WELCOME T

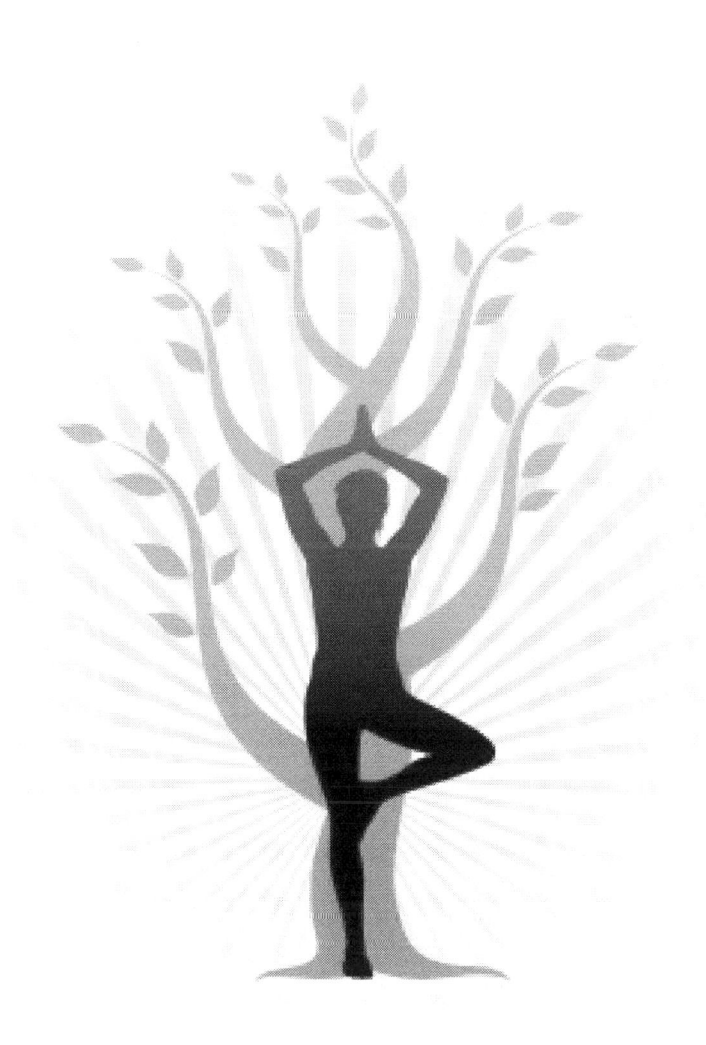

Knee Pain Recipe

KNEE PAIN RECIPE

The Ultimate Ingredients To Relieve Knee Pain Step-By-Step

Renee Moten

Text © by Renee Moten, 2018

PERSONAL DISCLAIMER

I am not a medical doctor. The information I provide is based on my personal experience as a Myoskeletal Therapist, Certified Personal Trainer & Massage Therapist. Any recommendations I made about weight training, alternative medicine or lifestyle should be discussed between you and your doctor.

Your results may vary with any of the following programs, and will be based on individual capacity, previous experience, ability to take action and varying level of desire. There are no guarantees concerning the level of success you may experience. Each individual's success depends on his or her background, dedication, desire and motivation.

All right reserved

No part of this publication may be reproduced to transmit in any form by any means, including photocopying, recording in any information storage and retrieval system, without the permission of the author except in the case of brief quotations embodied in critical articles or book reviews

I dedicate this book to my family, friends and especially my clients who have been patient and supportive as I sharpen my skills to become a holistic practitioner. Their invaluable physical participation and feedback has contributed greatly to the educational information in this book.

Future Vision

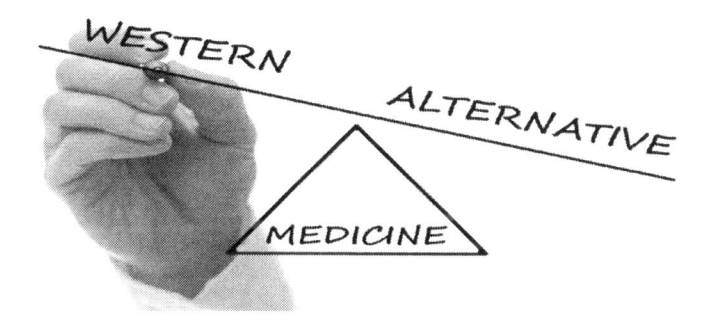

My vision is to one day see orthopedic doctors and alternative medicine practitioners' work together to create a therapy that can heal knee pain. An orthopedic doctor treats the painful knee with pharmaceuticals, physical therapy, cortisone shots and sometimes surgery. An alternative medicine practitioner treats knee pain by first realigning the body using stretching techniques, then using holistic methods to heal and relieve knee pain. Alternative practitioners and orthopedic doctors' strive to accomplish the same result of lessening the knee pain for the patient. So why not work together for the benefit of the patient.

Table of Contents

Introduction

Chapter 1   My Painful Years……………………11

Chapter 2   Chronic Inflammation ………………13

Chapter 3   What Causes Knee Pain……………15

Chapter 4   My Aha Moment……………………18

Chapter 5   Dry Brushing……………………...19

Chapter 6   Muscle Guarding……………………21

Chapter 7   Hydrotherapy………………….…22

Chapter 8   Stability Exercise……………………26

Chapter 9   Knee Pain Recipe (Step by Step)…….27

Summary

Author Notes

Introduction

Over many years, I have been both a Personal Trainer and patient. Experiencing unbearable knee pain, I have seen the role that alternative medicine has played in my life and the lives of my clients.

After participating in over 20,000 one-on-one training sessions as a Personal Trainer, I have created my own philosophy about the role doctors play in the treatment of chronic pain. Traditionally, the doctor's word was considered the final authority and went unquestioned. Alternative medicine is a viable option for my clients, but they do not even know that it is an option that could yield a mind blowing result. For centuries many people my clients inclusive, assume wrongly that prescription medication and surgery was the only way to relieve knee pain.

The reason behind me writing this publication is to encourage individuals to take immediate action when they are experiencing the first signs of knee pain. Even more importantly, when patients seek treatment, it is vital to know that there are other results-oriented actions to take aside from medication, shots or surgery. By acting quickly with full knowledge of their options, individuals can avoid further injury and a further complete breakdown of the knee cartilage or worse the pain of a "bone on bone" diagnosis.

Do not be afraid to look outside the box of western medicine. With applied knowledge comes the choice to find the treatment plan, which truly allows you to be both proactive and informed about your health.

Chapter 1

My Story "Many years of pain"

The spring of 1990, was when I first experienced a sharp pain in my right knee. It felt as if though someone had laid a hot poker on the front of my knee. Despite the searing pain, I could not recall any reasons why my right knee should be hurting. I couldn't remember having any recent injuries at the time, and my days of wearing high heel shoes were traded in long ago for tennis shoes.

For many years, I worked as a floor supervisor in the printing and mailing industry, which required me to be on my feet 10 hours a day, 6 days a week. In 1988, I had my first experience with severe pain in both feet. Just as I got out of bed, I felt a knife stabbing pain on both heels. I crawled to the phone to call a podiatrist. After speaking with a doctor, I was diagnosed with plantar fasciitis. The only remedy he offered was taping my arches and suggesting a cortisone shot, which I rejected. Although I was fitted with orthotics, my discomfort continued.

As someone who enjoyed sports and wanted to remain active, I refused to slow down. I limped around with my sore feet for three and a half years. Then during a 1990 exercise class, I experienced a sharp pain in my right knee. After going to the doctors, I was this time diagnosed with chondromalacia patella (patellofemoral syndrome), which he recommended treating with large doses of anti-inflammatory drugs and of course a cortisone shot. Despite the new diagnosis, I maintained my strong belief that I would only treat my pain with natural alternatives. Over the next 10 years, I went to 4 different orthopedic doctors, and each tried to treat me with cortisone shots, glucosamine, anti-inflammatory drugs, Synvisc Injections, and Celebrex. I said no to all of their recommendations. I continued on my journey in finding an answer, so I kept looking for natural remedies. Then it wasn't until 2001, that I finally experienced a breakthrough. After attending a fitness workshop, I learned that most knee pain is a result of **poor ankle rotation**, which leads me to my biggest realization.

    While playing soccer in the 1980's I suffered a fall which badly sprained my right ankle. Though I didn't experience any chronic ankle pain, the results of the injury eventually did impact my life and led me to write this publication. I hope that through my journey others can find their voice to speak up, and know that there are other options besides medication and surgical interventions.

Chapter 2

Chronic Pain

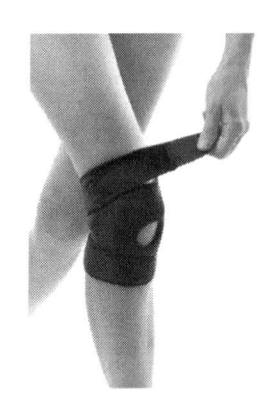

Beginning in the spring of 1991, I began to experience swelling and soreness in my right knee. Ice, heat and wearing a leg brace became my best friend. However, being a personal trainer, I thought that I could perform low impact exercises that would not irritate my knee. I was hopeful that by walking on the treadmill I could maintain a low impact workout and spare myself knee pain. But within a few minutes of walking on the treadmill, I knew that this plan was not going to work. Each walking step felt like my knees were bleeding inside, the soreness and stiffness were shaping into an explosion of pain. I did not stop walking I started to cry and wondered how I was going to continue exercising when I could not walk on a soft surface for few minutes. After all my years of being active, I felt defeated.

The pain I was experiencing in my knee I later discovered was caused by **inflammation.** It's an immune system response, which is a localized physical condition where part of the body becomes reddened, swollen, and hot and often results in severe pain. Initially, inflammation is beneficial to the injured knee. Once the body has fought off the invader and healed the damaged area, the symptoms of inflammation should subside — until the next time a joint gets damaged from injury or arthritis. When the incorrect therapy is used to reduce inflammation the person can experience pain for years and years.

The source of my knee pain <u>originated</u> from a sprained ankle during that soccer game in the 1980's. Poorly rotating ankles caused a slight limp in my walking gait. Eventually after years of limping both knees started to hurt. This went on to cause an immune system response, which initiated the production of inflammation that lasted for many years'.

Chapter 3

Causes of Knee Pain

There are many causes and treatments to alleviate knee pain. However, all knee pain has one key element in common. That is **inflammation**!! When you have chronic inflammation, your body's inflammatory response can eventually start damaging healthy cells, tissues, and organs. It's next to impossible to heal knee pain without first addressing the persistence inflammation response.

1. **Twisting your Ankle:** over time pain usually starts on the outside of the knee.
2. **Tendinitis:** pain in the front of the knee that is made worse when climbing, taking stairs, or walking up an incline.
3. **Bursitis:** inflammation caused by repeated overuse or injury of the knee.
4. **Chondromalacia** patella: damaged cartilage under the kneecap. gout: arthritis caused by the buildup of uric acid
5. **Meniscus tear:** a tear in the knee cartilage is a common injury, and typically requires surgery.

6. **What are the bottoms of your shoes telling you?** Most people don't know it, but the wear pattern on a well-used pair of shoes can tell a pretty good story. Pronation and Supination are natural, normal motions of the foot. The problem tends to be when someone pronates and supinates too much. This places extra stress on the foot and can result in running and walking incurred injuries, such as iliotibial band syndrome of the knee. Below are examples of over pronation and over supination.

Supination (outward rolling) places an enormous strain on the muscles and tendons that stabilize the ankle. Constant walking or running can lead to the ankle rolling, thereby causing knee pain and ankle strains.

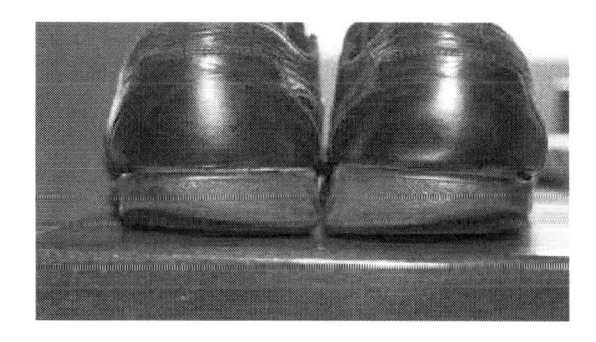

Pronation is the inward movement of the foot as it rolls to distribute the force of impact off the ground as you run. This movement is critical to proper shock absorption. When excessive pronation occurs, the foot arch flattens out and stretches the muscles, tendons and ligaments underneath the foot. Continue flattening of the arches adds stress to the knee joint creating an inflammation response and pain.

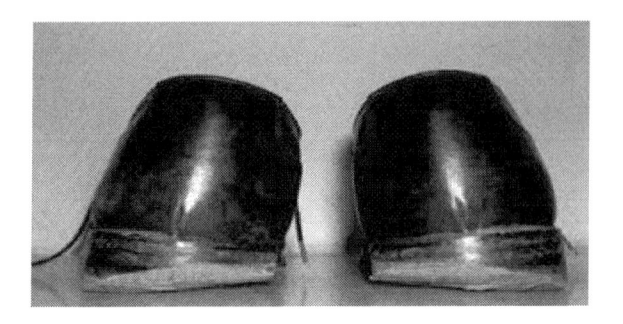

Chapter 4

My Aha Moment

I decided after visiting 4 orthopedic doctors that I would use alternative medicine to heal my knee pain. I've learned over the years what techniques work and that which does not work. You are very fortunate to have this book. Without doubt, I can say there is no other pain management protocol that comes close to relieving knee pain without drugs and shots like Knee Pain Recipe.

The following pages will take you through an incredibly easy process of techniques and instructions. The only requirement is that you be patient and enjoy the process.

Chapter 5

Dry Brushing and the Lymphatic System

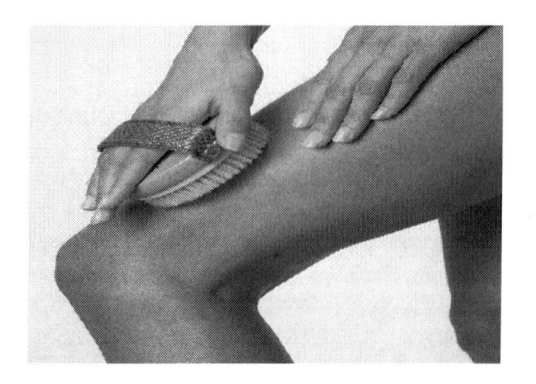

In the 1990's I first learned about exfoliation through an introduction to dry brushing. Our skin breathes! Dry skin brushing increases circulation to the skin, thereby encouraging our body's discharge of metabolic wastes. Then there is an increased blood flow that begins to enter the areas brushed, as you will experience an increase in electromagnetic energy that helps you to feel energized and invigorated. You will start by using a soft bristle brush to brush towards the heart, and starting at the toe then ending at the head.

I began using the dry brush technique as a monthly practice. So, as I continued on my journey to finding a holistic methods of pain relief, I noticed that on certain days my knee pain would lessen after the brushing. Feeling excited about this discovery, I began to seek more information concerning exfoliation. That information led me to discover MLD.

    I learned about Manual Lymphatic Drainage (MLD) after receiving my first pedicure in 2004; MLD is a type of gentle massage, which is intended to encourage the natural drainage of lymph, which is a clear-to-white solution made of white blood cells and fluids from the intestine. When the lymphatic system gets **congested** with waste and metabolic toxin participles, the buildup has the potential to make a person sick. Inflammation and disease are often a result of **lymphatic congestion.** Arthritis has the potential to cause the build-up of metabolic toxic wastes, which can lead to painful knees.

Chapter 6

What is Muscle Guarding?

Muscle guarding is a protective response in muscles that results from pain and the fear of movement. While I was managing my pain, I noticed that there were many mornings where I was unable to straighten my knees completely; and even in the simple task of rising from a chair, or going up and down stairs caused excruciating pain. I started feeling old before my time.

After extensive research, I found out that I was experiencing muscle guarding. My body was trying to protect the painful knee joint from movement by tightening the muscles around my knee to prevent the joints from being re-injured. To regain muscle flexibility a stretching regimen was necessary to bring blood flow and oxygen to the tightened muscles. I began **stretching** each morning, and almost overnight the morning stiffness lessened. Muscle guarding and dysfunction are a cycle, which when left unbroken can lead to spasms and chronic pain for years.

Chapter 7

Hydrotherapy - Healing with Water

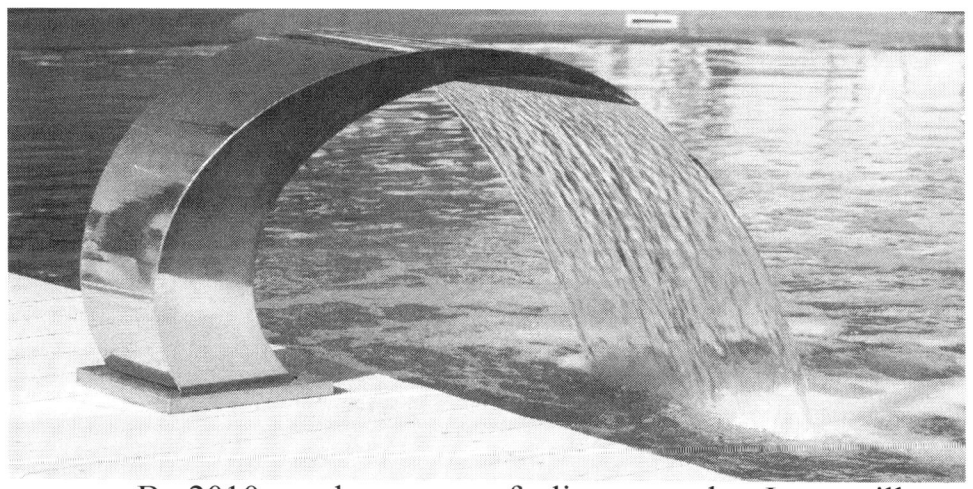

By 2010, my knees were feeling great, but I was still experiencing occasional flare-ups of residual pain. It was amazing to later find out that a solution was right in front of me, and I never considered it. This was a simple solution of hydrotherapy.

Hydrotherapy is just as simple as it sounds; it is a therapy that uses the healing powers of water. To receive the full benefits of hydrotherapy you have to use cold water, so brace yourself to be a little chilly. The process itself is very simple.

Cold showers or alternating shower temperatures between warm and cold has a powerful effect on circulation. When you expose yourself to cold temperatures, your body constricts blood supply. When exposed to heat the vessels dilate and expand. Changing these temperatures and using cold water dramatically improves the tone of the blood vessel walls. This gives the body greater adaptability in driving blood into areas that are needed.

This also dramatically improves lymphatic flow. The lymph system carries away waste products from immune-related activity. Lymphatic flow depends upon muscle contraction to move through the system. If the lymphatic flow is slow or stagnant, it leads to pooling and lymph edema in the lower extremities.

As with any treatment plan, consistency is the only way to see results. I began by using hydrotherapy 4 days in a row, twice a day. The relief I experienced was miraculous. I was in such disbelief I decided to put my knees to the ultimate test by entering two 5k races in 2012. Once I finished both of those races with minimal knee discomfort I decided to conquer the Avon 40 mile walk.

Not only did I finish the race within the time limit, aside from a small blister, I also experienced no knee discomfort. It was such a feeling of accomplishment to finish the race, but even more when I realized how far I had come from crying on the treadmill to walking 40 miles with no knee pain. It took time and a lot of patience, but in the end I found relief on my own terms

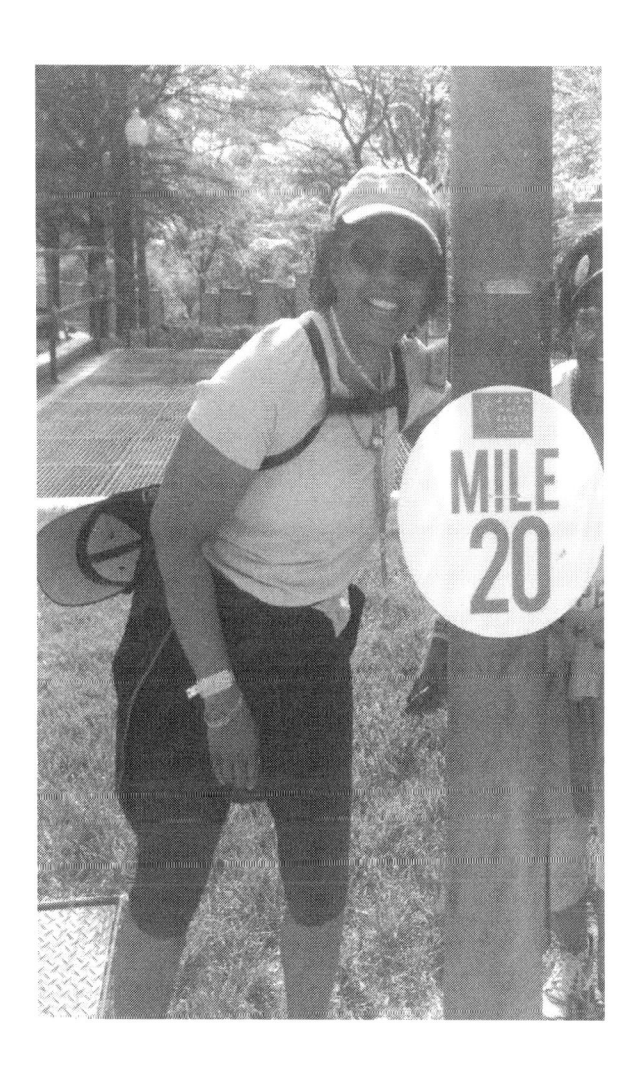

Chapter 8

Exercise and Stability Training

When a person is experiencing physical pain, the idea of strength training can be considered impossible. Unfortunately, knee pain often results in weakness in the legs. In order to graduate back into a more active lifestyle, it is important to recreate muscle balance throughout the body.

Where to start? Not all exercises are actually helpful in relieving knee pain. In fact, if you are not careful attempting strength training, you can actually cause additional damages and an inflammation response. After years of using exercises prescribed by a physical therapist, doctors and friends, I realized that trying to strengthen muscles that are tight and attached to **inflamed joints** is like a person trying to canoe upstream without a paddle. You will never get to your destination.

If you do not first address the inflammation around the joint, then you will be unable to stabilize the joint, strengthen the muscles and relieve your pain. **Strength training is not recommended when your knees are in pain.**

Chapter 9

Knee Pain Recipe

Well you've made it to the most important page. Now let's relieve the pain in your knees in the next couple of days.

You **must** follow the steps in this order:

Step 1	Dry Brushing
Step 2	Hydrotherapy
Step 3	Lymphatic Drainage
Step 4	Muscles Guarding/ Stretching
Step 5	Chiropractic alignment
Step 6	Stability& Strengthening Exercises

Note: This program works 90% of the time. People, who are taking anti-inflammatory drugs, have had arthroscopic surgery or a knee replacement may have a bigger challenge getting rid of the pain.

The following pages will give you a step by step instruction on how to perform The Knee Pain Recipe.

Step 1

Dry Brushing

You have swelling because your knee lives in a toxic, inflammatory environment. Dry brushing will detox the knee.

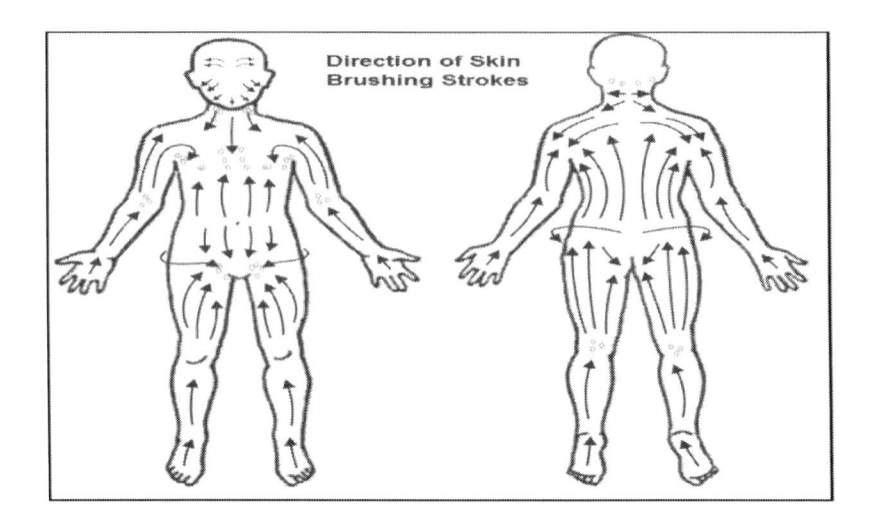

How to Dry Brush:

1. Use a natural soft bristle brush. They can be found at any health food store. Cost: about $20.
2. Dry brush using the chart as your guide. You will be sloughing off some serious dry skin. After brushing proceed to the shower and perform hydrotherapy.
3. Avoid sensitive areas like bruises, and anywhere the skin is broken, such as areas of skin rash, wounds, cuts or infections. Also never brush an area affected by poison oak, poison ivy or sunburn.

4. The entire body should be brushed, including your back, but skip the face and scalp (and maybe breasts). Use long sweeping strokes starting from the bottom of your feet upwards, and from the hands towards the shoulders, and on the torso in an upward direction to help drain the lymph back towards your heart.
5. Use the amount of pressure that is right for you; at the beginning, always thread on the side of caution
6. Take your time and do it right; dry brushing should take 7-12 minutes,

Perform this ritual: 3 times a week for 2 weeks

Step 2

Hydrotherapy

Hydrotherapy shuts down the inflammation to stop joint erosion.

How to Perform Hydrotherapy

I: Step into the shower turn on the hot water. Allow the water to run for about 1 minute, paying special attention to make sure that you're sore joints are feeling the warmth of the water. Using a shower wand (if available) spray the water directly on the sore joints.

II: After the 1 minute of hot water, quickly turn the water to cold and allow it to run for 30 seconds. Though the cold water is shocking it is the only way to receive the full benefits of hydrotherapy.

III: Repeat interchanging the hot and cold 5 times per shower. That's it. You will feel pain relief within a matter of days.

The reason this process works so well is that the hot water stimulates blood flow to the surface of the body, while cold water stimulates blood flow to the core of the body.

Perform this ritual: 2 times a day for 2 weeks

Note: Immersing your whole body in the ritual can give a person tremendous benefits. Brrr!!

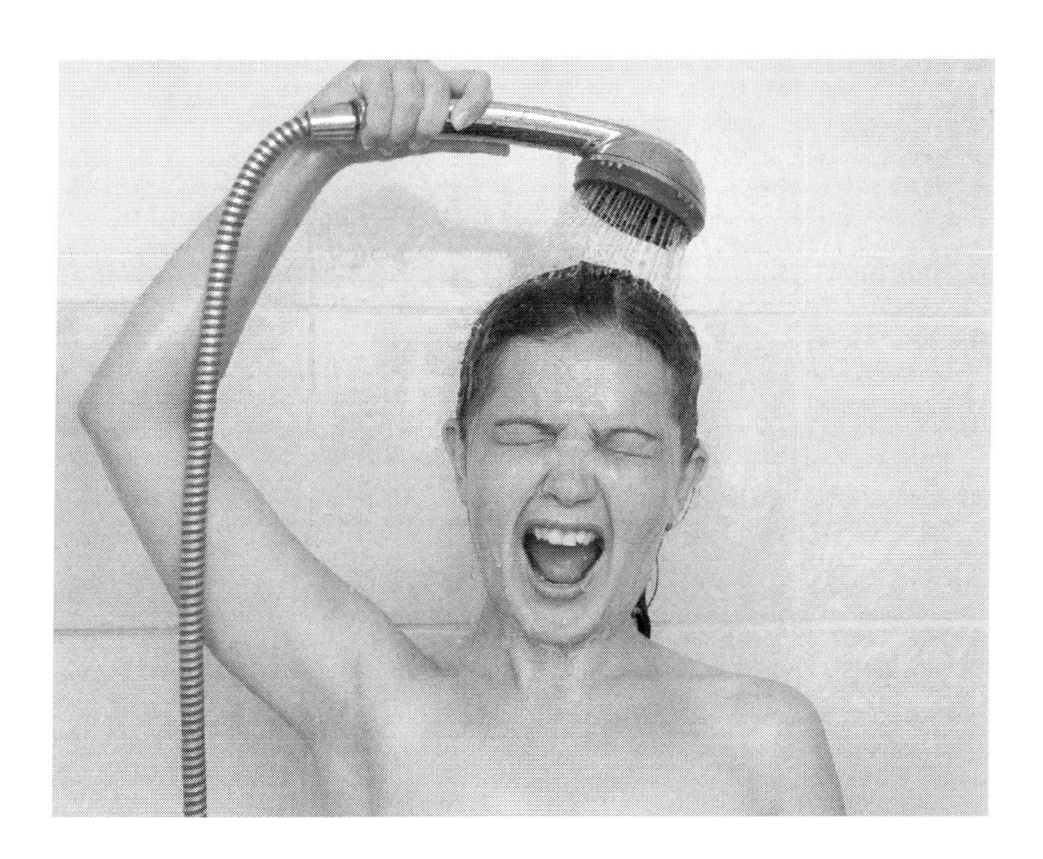

Step 3

Lymphatic Drainage Massage

Lymphatic Massage reduces the stiffness in painful knees. Hiring a massage therapist is needed for this part.

Manual Lymphatic Drainage (MLD) benefits are numerous and include; clearing areas of congestion such as swollen ankles, puffy eyes and swollen legs. Manual lymph drainage is a type of gentle massage which is intended to encourage the natural drainage of lymph, which carries waste products away from the tissue back to the heart.

Perform MLD: 2 times in one month. In the second month, you will begin reflexology and trigger point therapy.

Step 4

Muscle Guarding/ Stretching

Stretching brings the back range of motion within the body

These six stretches on the following pages *must* be done every day for 2 to 3 weeks along with steps 1 through 3. Once your flexibility has returned and knee pain lessens stability training becomes the next step.

Performing the proper stretches in the <u>appropriate order</u> is crucial to the success of holistically rehabilitating your knees.

1. Foot circles
2. Tennis ball rolling
3. Calf Stretch
4. Shin Stretch
5. Hamstring stretch
6. Quadriceps Stretch

IMPORTANT: As you continue to stretch daily keep a log of which leg is becoming more flexible. Muscle imbalance is one of the major causes of knee pain. Improving flexibility in both legs is the goal of the stretching regimen.

Ankle circles <u>must</u> be done first.

Performing ankle circles loosens the muscles and tendons in the leg and the joint around the foot. Stiffness in the ankles can lead to stress in the foot and the legs, leading to knee pain, back pain, and neck pain.

Action: Point your toes at the ceiling in a ballerina pose, and then slowly start to rotate the foot in a full circle. Rotate the foot without moving the leg, so that the entire rotation is taking place in the joint of the ankle

Perform 30 reps to the left. 30 reps going to the right. Repeat on both feet

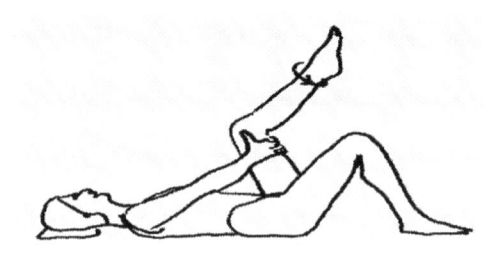

Continue for 3 weeks (This may be painful. Stop and rest then proceed again. Don't give up they will loosen up)

Tennis Ball Rolling

"Gait" means the way a person walks. Abnormal gait or gait abnormality occurs when the body systems that control the way a person walks do not function in the usual way. Most people may not feel pain or soreness in their feet. From experience, I've found that if you have knee pain, your feet and ankles become sore and stiff, thereby contributing to the misalignment of the knee joint and cause more pain. Tennis ball rolling relieves the tension in the ligaments and muscles on the bottom of your feet stimulating blood flow in the area.

Sit on the edge of a chair or stand with a tennis ball under your arch. Roll the ball around in small circles, with the ball under your foot. This process may be painful, but keep rolling every day until the pain has subsided.

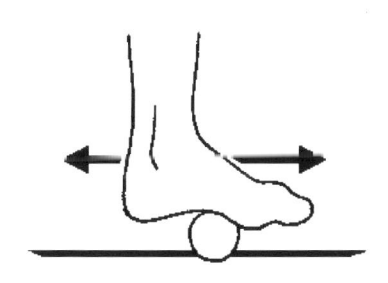

Calf Stretch

Tightness in your calf muscles can be one cause of knee pain. Your calf muscles may require improved flexibility if you have an injury or illness that prevents normal mobility. By working to keep your calf muscles flexible, you can get back to moving normally. Pull toes to the ceiling and hold for 5 to 7 seconds.

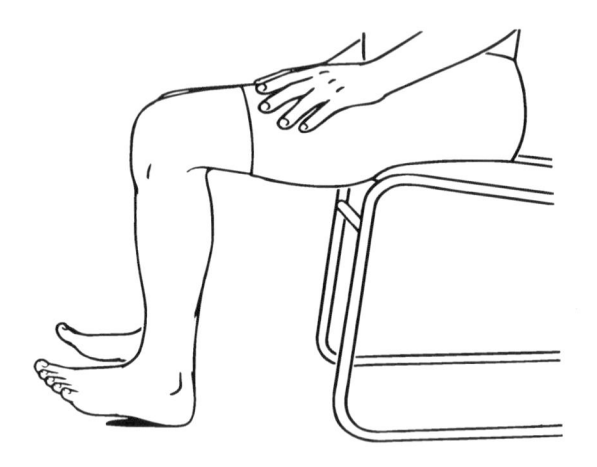

Perform stretch hold for 5 to 7 seconds. Repeat 10 reps daily for 3 weeks. Continue until a stretch is no longer felt in the calf. Then proceed to a standing calf stretch.

Shin Stretch

The anterior tibialis muscle (Shins) lifts your toes off the ground – it is an important movement for climbing stairs and walking uphill. These muscles also play an important role in maintaining your balance. Stretching this muscle will usually cause a cramp in the calf so be prepared. Stop the stretch let the calf calm down then try again.

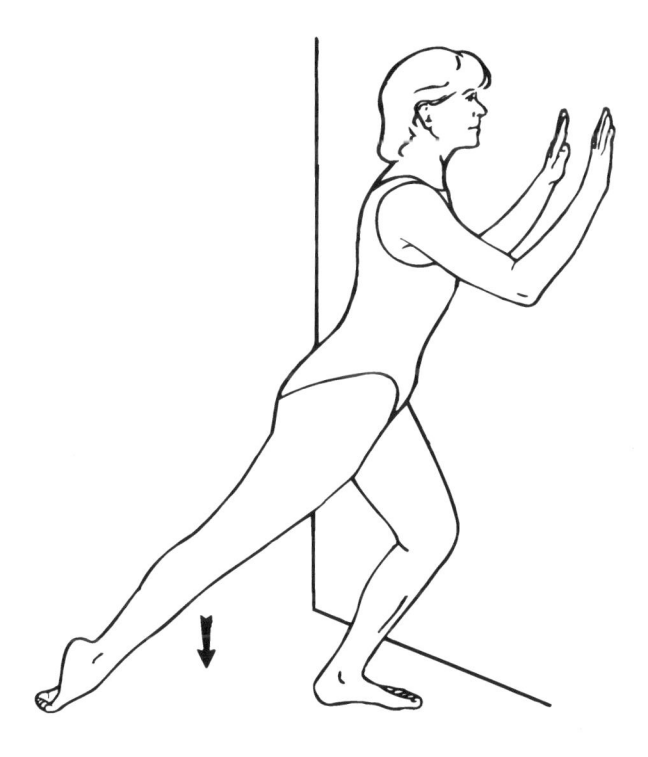

Perform stretch hold for 5 to 7 seconds. Repeat 5 reps daily for 3 weeks.

Hamstring Stretch

Lie down on your back and place a towel or strap around the ball of your foot. Hold the strap/towel on each end and straighten your leg towards the ceiling. Pull your leg, with the towel/ strap towards your chest for 10 reps hold for 5 to 7 seconds and then switch the legs and repeat the same procedure.

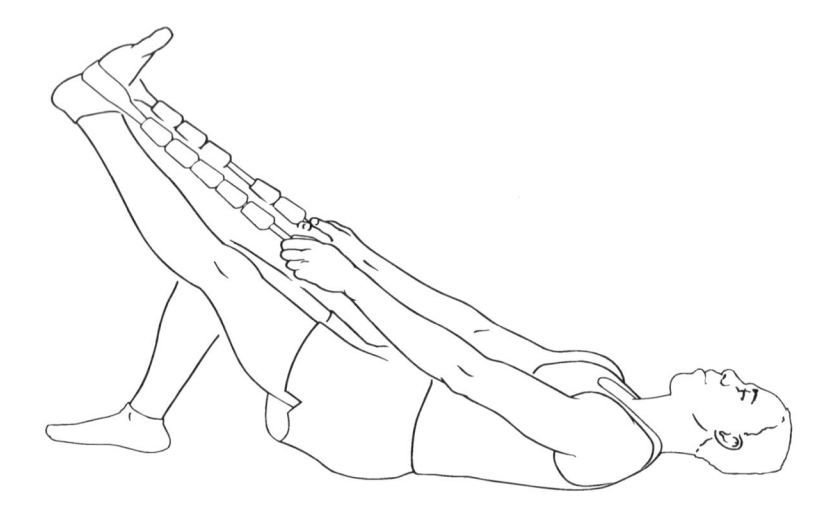

Perform stretch hold for 5 to 7 seconds. Repeat 10 reps daily for 3 week. (As you're stretching push your heel to the ceiling. This may be a little painful)

Lying Quadriceps Stretch

Lie on your side and rest your head on one hand. Keep your knees together and gently pull your right heel towards the buttocks until a stretch is felt in the front thigh (quadriceps or 'quads'). (If unable to grab ankle use a towel)

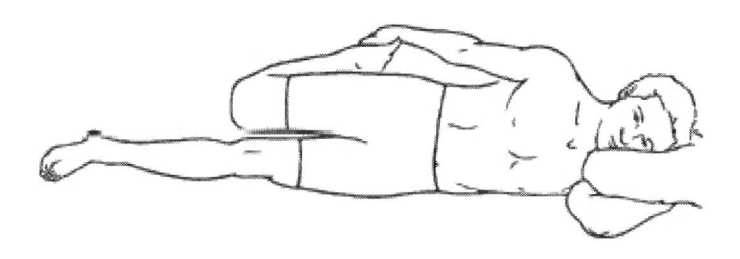

Perform daily stretch hold for 5 to 7 seconds. Repeat 5 reps for 3 weeks.

Step 5

Hiring an Applied Kinesiology Chiropractor

Feet, ankle, hip and back must be in alignment before starting exercises

What is Applied Kinesiology?

It's a manual method that assesses structural, chemical and mental aspects of health using manual muscle testing, combined with other standard methods of diagnosis. Applied Kinesiology gives the doctor added ability to evaluate the function of the nervous system, which controls the organs, glands, and other tissues.

First visit – Ankles, toes, hips and feet must be adjusted
Adrenals, liver and thyroid must be muscle tested for strength
Second visit – Adductors, Abductors, Gluteus Muscles and Quads must be adjusted
Adrenals, liver, spleen, kidneys and pituitary gland must be muscle tested for strength
Third visit – Re-check all the above organs and muscles then proceed to the upper body.

Step 6

Stabilizing & Strengthening Exercises

Proper Alignment Reduces Pain

The soft tissues of the body (muscles, tendons, ligaments, etc.) help maintain proper alignment of the bones during movement. If bones aren't properly aligned when they move through a range of motion, there can be a great deal of friction, a lack of stability, decreased mobility and compromised function.

The best way to maintain biomechanical integrity during movement is with the proper balance of strength and flexibility training. Muscles work in pairs (extensors and flexors) and maintaining the proper balance of strength in these muscle pairs can go a long way to prevent joint pain and injury.

Many exercises can be used in this section. I will introduce three I find the most helpful.

Note: To learn more about the correct exercises contact kneepainrecipe@gmail.com

Exercise: Sit and Stand/<u>add a pillow</u> to the chair seat if needed

Action: The person sits with the knees bent and feet directly under the knees. In a slow and controlled manner, the person moves from a seated position to standing and then back to a seated position as shown. To ensure the knees do not fall inward add a pillow or small ball between the knees to maintain alignment.

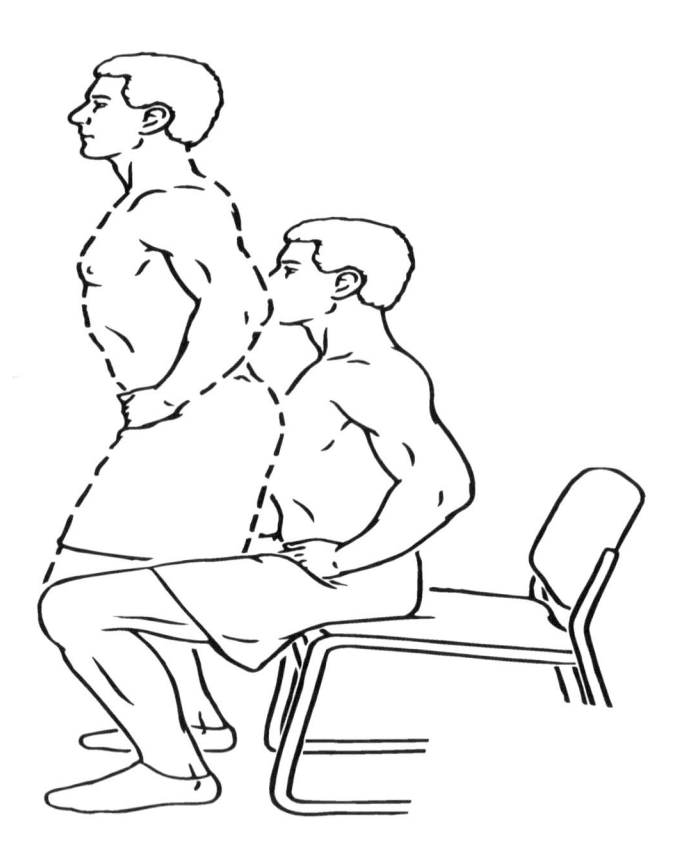

Perform Exercise: 30 Reps 4 days a week for 3 weeks.

Exercise: The Clam

Action: Lie on your side on the floor with your legs together, knees bent and with your head, shoulders, hip and heels touching the floor. Open your top knee towards the roof to full rotation while keeping the heels connected.

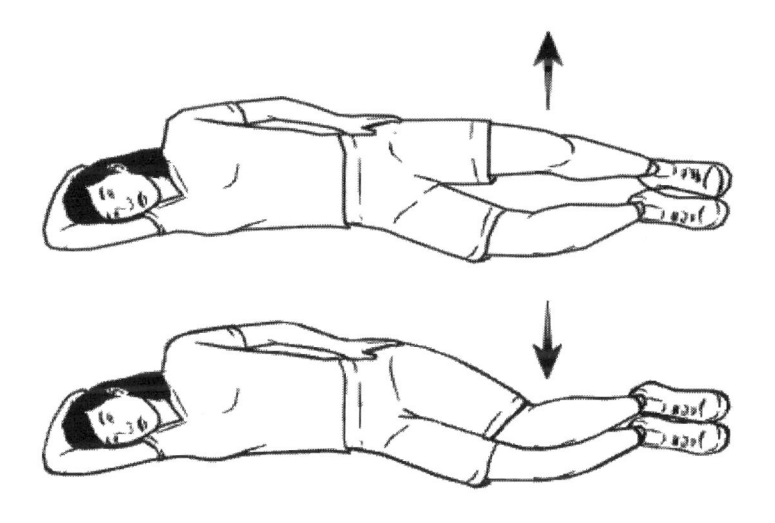

Perform Exercise: 30 Reps 4 days a week for 3 weeks.

Exercise: Pillow Squeeze (Isometric Adduction)

With a ball or bended pillow between your knees squeeze the knees together hold for 20 seconds. Lie down or come up onto your elbows.

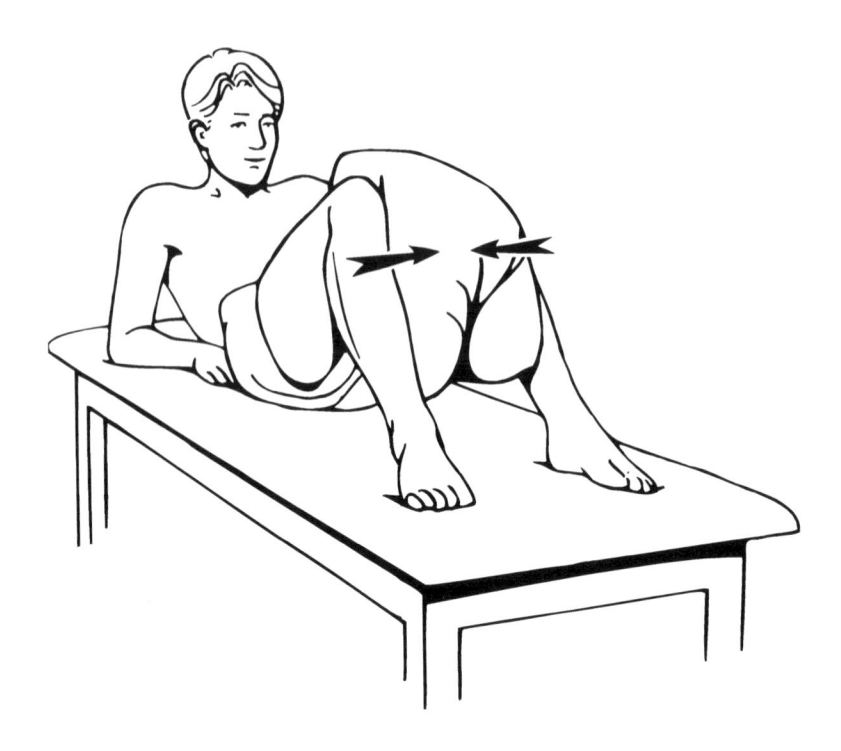

Perform Exercise: Hold for 20 seconds and release.

Repeat 8 Reps every day for 2 weeks

Knee Replacement Statics

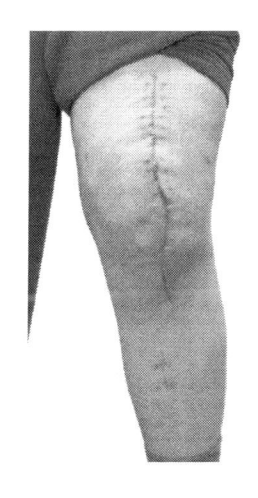

More than 600,000 knee replacements are performed each year in the United States. With an aging population staying in the workforce longer and obesity on the rise, demand for total knee replacement surgery is expected to exceed 3 million by the year 2030.

The average hospital charge for a total knee replacement (TKR) in the United States is $49,500. Medicare recently reported that in 2014, it paid for more than 400,000 of these operations, which cost more than $7 billion for the hospitalizations alone. The average cost for these procedures, including hospitalization and recovery, ranged from $16,500 to $33,000, depending on geographic location. Wow, the cost is staggering.

The Knee Pain Recipe doesn't leave a scar and costs about $200 total. It does not require an operation, cortisone shot, medication or physical therapy. It just needs patience, and a desire to heal the body using alternative methods'.

Summary

Knee Pain Recipe requires no drugs, no surgery and no traveling to a physical therapist twice a week. The only requirement is your desire, commitment and discipline to step outside the box of medical science and use the tools that nature has given you to heal your body. Each of us is truly in charge of taking back control of our health. Knee Pain Recipe gives you a choice between alternative medicine and western medicine. The more we work with our bodies, by giving it truly what it needs to heal, the less we will need to resort to treatments that do not work.

    Namaste

Notes from the Author

Renee Moten once felt pain in both knees for many years. Determined to heal her knees using natural techniques has allowed her to become educated in the holistic world of pain relief.

She has become a sought-after fitness professional on the east coast and an undisputed trendsetter and leader in her field. She has personally helped many people relieve knee pain through her programs of teaching them to nutritionally nourish their bodies, while helping them learn the ways of living a holistic healthy life.

In Renee Moten's Knee Pain Recipe she shares her secrets on how to take back control of your health using techniques that have been around for centuries. She provides information about what the body needs in order to heal itself and relieve pain.

Kneepainrecipe@gmail.com

https://www.facebook.com/kneepaincoach

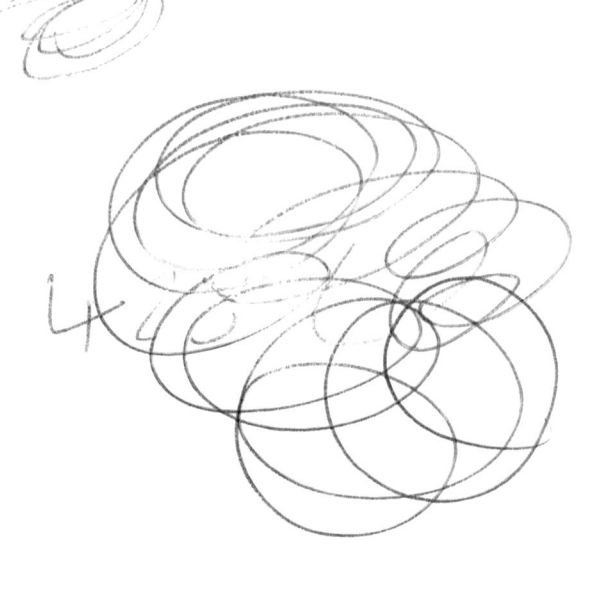

$$
\begin{array}{r}
428 \\
289 \\
1099 \\
\underline{}\\
1816 \\
1230 \\
3046 \\
\underline{}\\
3552
\end{array}
$$

$$
\begin{array}{r}
3046 \\
750 \\
\hline
3796
\end{array}
$$